I0467769

Fore Word

The book is intended for persons who have a noise problem, want to know what is causing the noise, and where it comes from.

Once this is known most maintenance persons will be able to work out how to eliminate the problem.

10 years ago I started using laptop computers and good quality microphones to detect and eliminate noise hazards.

The price of the instrument was measured in the thousands of dollars.

5 Years ago I started using video technology to overcome some of the limitations of walking around with a laptop.

Now smartphones will do most of what I was doing 10 years ago with expensive equipment, and most of what I was doing with video.

This book will show you how to use a Smartphone to detect noise.

- Choosing Microphones
- Using microphones
- Calibrating Smartphones
- dB Apps
- Spectrum analyser Apps

Once detected and measured noise can then be eliminated.

Another of my books "Eliminate noise Hazards" can be used with this book.

TABLE OF CONTENTS

1.0 Basic Principles

- Noise gets louder as we get closer to the source
- Noise gets quieter as we move away
- Point towards the source it gets louder
- Point away it gets softer.
- Flat surfaces radiate noise and it may be difficult to determine the exact source.
- Ears are not always the best measurement tool.

If these principles are understood then most sources of noise can be located.

What we need is a means to measure.

Smartphones can be used to measure.

2.0 Smartphones as measurement tools

Smartphones have a built in microphone. This microphone is biased towards human speech. It is biased to pick up sounds that are very close.
Measuring sound will always vary

- Readings will vary dependent upon what weighting scale is used i.e. a reading using the "A" scale will differ from that using the "D" scale using the same instrument in exactly the same position
- The type of microphone used to measure will also have an effect
- Moving a slightly in another direction can affect the reading.

In real terms

- We only need a fixed number for comparison.
- 75dB is problematic.
- 85dB and hearing protection should be worn.
- It does not matter if the reading is 86 or 87dB its just too loud.
- Our focus should be on reducing noise levels.

The purpose of measuring noise is so we have a hard numerical value against which we can measure improvements.

2.1 dB Apps

There are a number of Apps that turn the Smartphone into a dB meter.

These can be found in the Apps stores.

Most of these will be accurate enough to give an indication of noise levels.

Because the microphone in the cell phone is biased towards human speech, the apps have a bias towards human speech.

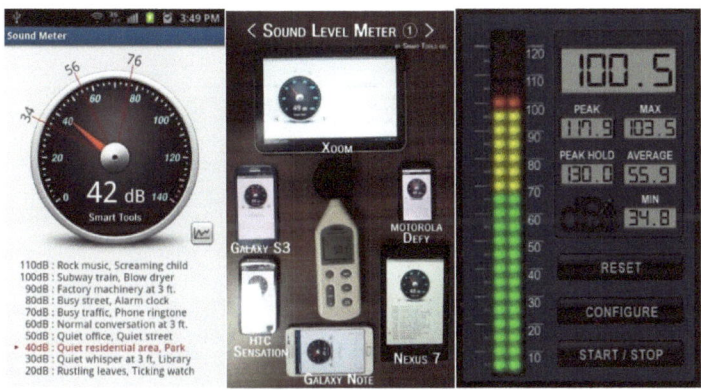

Most apps will be good enough to indicate if we have a problem

- Test the blow drier
- Test the lawn mower
- Test the TV

2.1.1 Calibrating an App

Calibrating is setting the instrument to give a true reading. If the instrument is reading high or low we can add or subtract from the actual reading
I.e. the app reads 92dB, the true reading is 90dB. Take 2 dB off the reading

- Install App
- Measure a known noise source with a dB meter
- Compare the dB meter with the Smartphone App

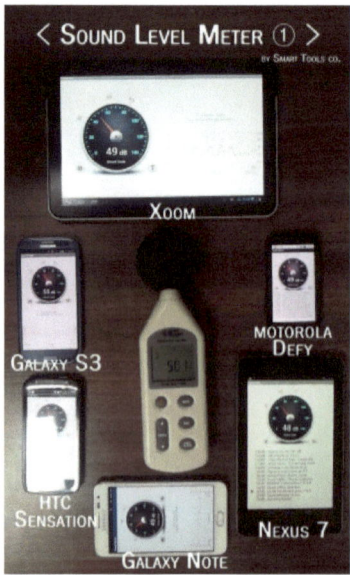

Some Apps store display the reading of the App against a dB meter.
If your smartphone is on the list you can tell if it reads high or low.

2.2 Spectrum analyser Apps

A spectrum analyser breaks the sound into individual frequencies.
This can be useful to detect resonance peaks.
It also can be used to indicate what type of sound is being produced.

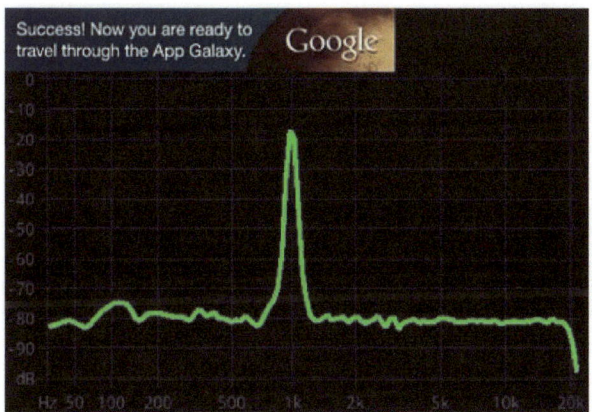

FrequenSee - Spectrum Analyzer
Daniel Bach- April 13, 2012

There are a number on the market.
I would suggest trying several till one that suits your phone is found.
Using a directional mic with an app can be highly effective in locating a particular sound. If we can locate the peak, then a significant lowering of noise can be achieved.

3.0 Microphones

The microphone built into the smartphone will work Ok. Upgrading the microphone will greatly improve the sound capabilities of the Smartphone. We can use the bias built into microphone to make picking up noise sources easier.

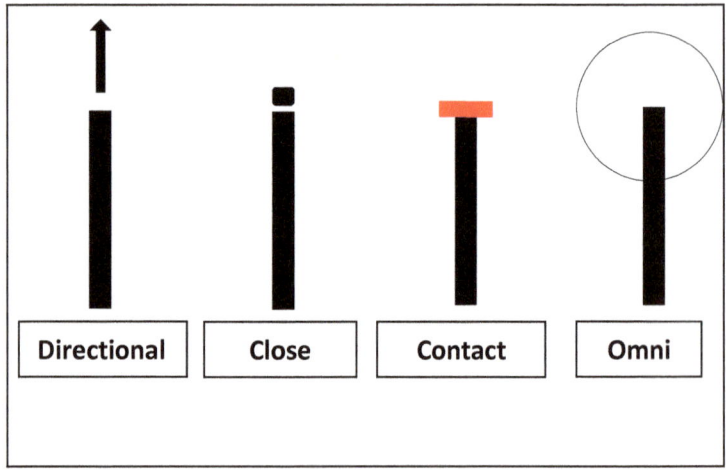

Directional mic

Use if we want to know the direction a noise is coming from.

Close

Use around machinery.

Contact Microphones

Use on surfaces where we suspect noise is being radiated via vibration.

Omni

Use to pick up all the sounds in a room for a general reading.

3.1 Directional Microphones

These detect noise in in a narrow beam facing forward. They are sometimes called shotgun microphones. They range in price from $20 -$2,000

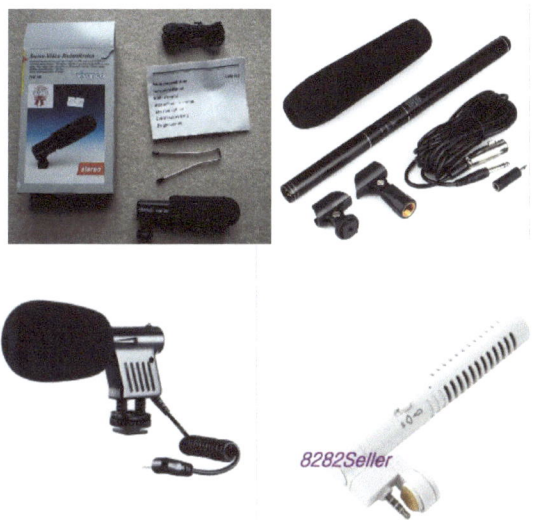

These are examples from on line stores.
Point the Microphone at the suspected noise source and the volume will increase. Point away and it will decrease.
These can be used with the video function of the smartphone
Plug a directional microphone into any device.
Noise will get louder when the device is pointed towards a sound source and quieter when pointed away.
It will get louder as you walk towardsthe sorce

It is not necessary to get exact dB readings.
The noise level will increase as one gets closer to the source.
Pointing towards or away from a source will also change the

3.1.1 Using Directional Microphones

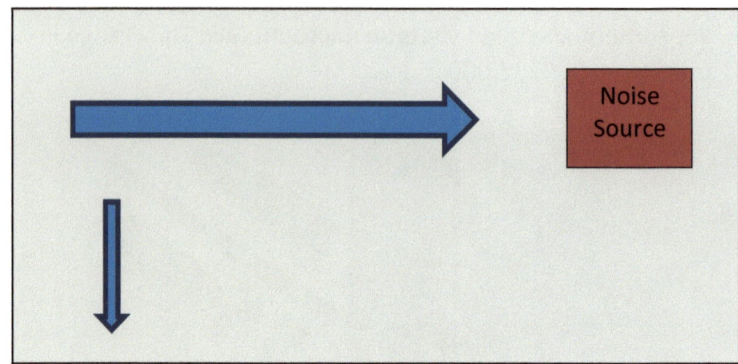

Pointing towards the source the noise gets louder
Pointing away it becomes quieter.

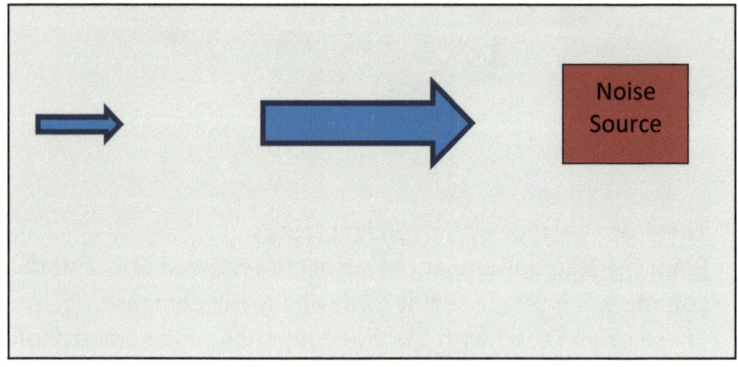

Noise becomes louder as we approach the source.

3.1.1 Directional Microphones with spectrum analysers.

This is a method to use when we wish to trace a particular frequency.

Often used when the noise is leaking from a room.

Particularly useful for environmental issues.

1/ Lock onto a peak

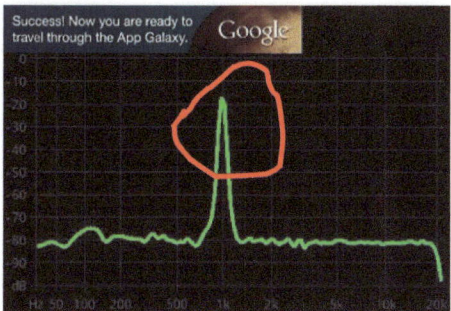

The peak will increase or decrease with direction and proximity.

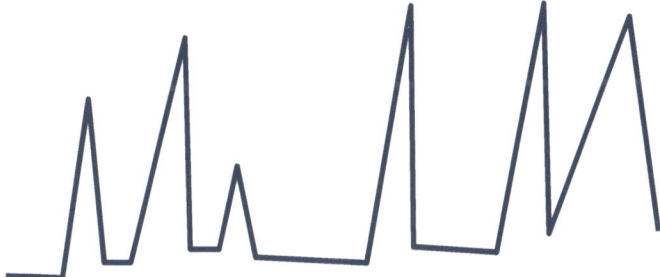

For Multiple peaks select one and focus on it.

3.2 Close Proximity Microphones (Vocal)

These were originally designed for bands. They will pick up sounds close to the singer much better than sounds further away. This is to prevent feedback or the high pitched squeal.

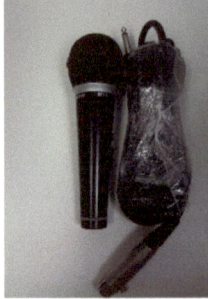 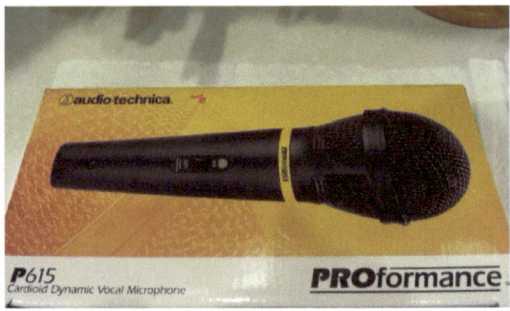

These can be plugged into any device.
They range in price from $10-$1,000
Avoid models that require batteries or phantom power

Search under vocal mics on any online store.

3.2.1 Using Close Microphones

1/ Move the microphone around the machine as it is running
2/ Locate areas where sound is louder
3/ Compare different operating conditions
4/ Taking a video for later analysis can be very helpful Compare
5/ Usually we would switch to a contact microphone to get a better idea of the cause and source

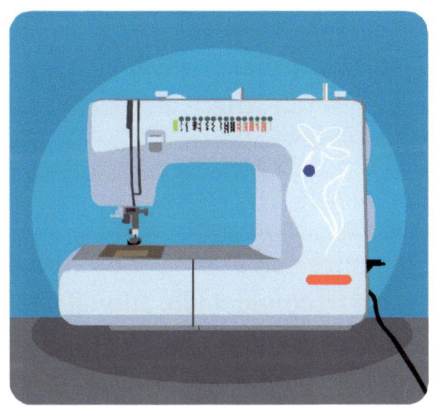

3.3 Contact Microphones

These will only pick up sound from a surface.
Sometimes they are called boundary microphones.
Very handy to detect noise from pipes or flat surfaces

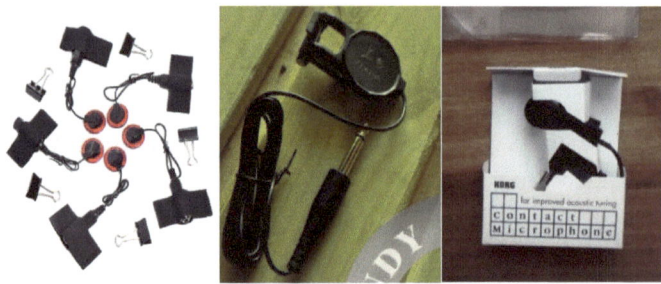

There are all sorts out there. It will be necessary to purchase an adapter, as there are very few made for smartphones.

Contact Microphones can also be used with spectrum analyser software to conduct vibrational analysis.

3.3.1 Using Contact Mics

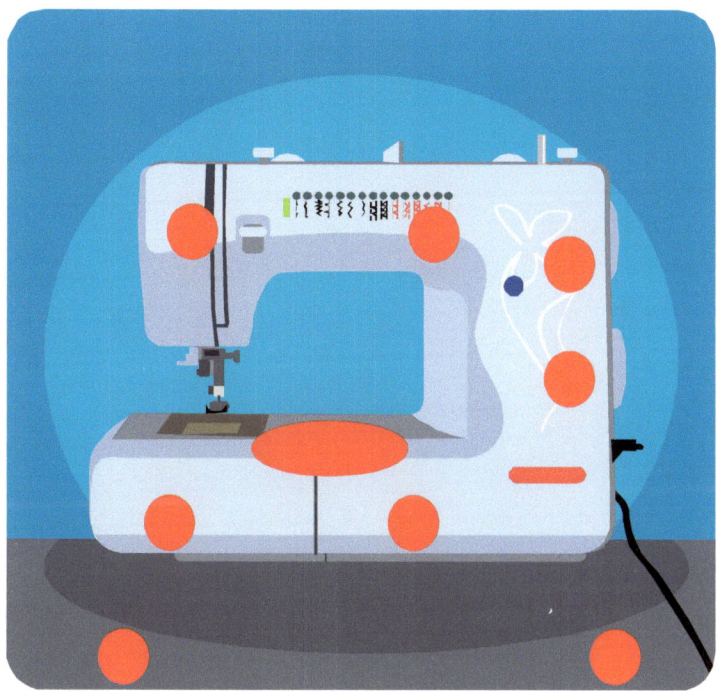

1/Take readings all around the machine.
2/Make changes and measure
3/ What is the effect?
4/ Measure what the machine is sitting on. Often the source from the stand or floor is greater than that of the machine.

> If we have similar machines, take measurements form each and compare.
> What is different?

3.4 Omi Directional Microphones

These pick up sound from all around the microphone. Generally they pick up room ambience.

4.0 Connecting microphones to a smartphone.

There are an increasing number of microphones made specifically for smartphones. These plug directly into the phone.
It is preferable to get one that is made specifically for your phone.
There can be issues with matching the power of the Microphone to the input of the phone

Search online for
"Microphones for cell phones
"Microphones for smartphones"
"Microphones for iPhone "

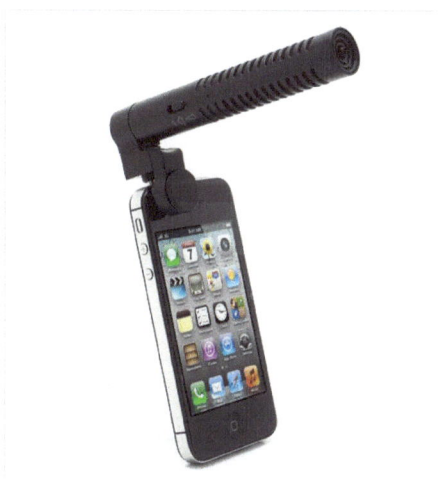

If an adapter is needed
Search You Tube for
 "External Microphone for smartphone "
Or Microphone adapter for (Brand name of Phone)

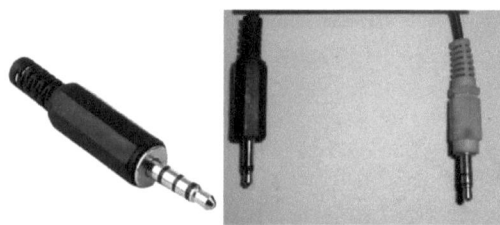

Plugging a microphone directly into a smartphone will not work. It needs the plug on the left to disable the internal mic of the smartphone.
When the plug is removed the mic in the smart phone will become active again.
The type of plug needed will vary between makes of phone.

4.1 Wiring Diagram for adapter.

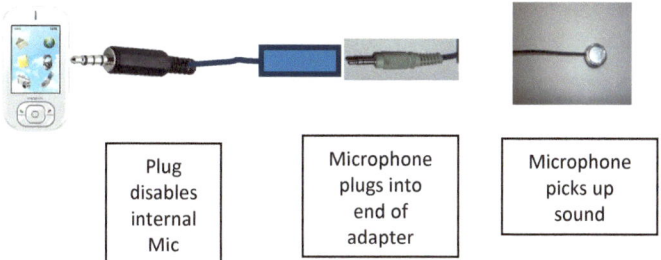

| Plug disables internal Mic | Microphone plugs into end of adapter | Microphone picks up sound |

5.0 Where to measure

5.1 Noise gets loader as we approach the source.

Generally the noise increases the closer we get to the source. There are a couple of traps.

- We may be approaching or leaving another source. It can be particularly difficult if there are flat surfaces or pipes that radiate sound.
- What we are measuring may not be the source.

5.2 Turn machines off and on-

- This may seem obvious but it can be overlooked. Turn the machine of and on. What is the difference?

5.3 Tighten anything that is loose

- This is a case of shooting on suspicion. May take longer to measure than it does to tighten.

5.4 Holes

- Any hole can act as an amplifier. This is true for cavities which amplify sound in the same way a guitar does.

5.5 Pipes on walls

- Be suspicious if a pipe is attached to a wall.
- When the pipe moves the wall can too.

5.6 Pipes attached to compressors and pumps
- It is not unusual for a pump or compressor to make noise.
- Often the source of the noise is the pipes and what is attached to the pump.
- Acoustic enclosures can be built. If the source of the noise is coming from the pipes the enclosure will be of limited value.

5.7 Handrails and railings
- Rollercoasters address noise, by filling pipes with sand. This dampens the noise made by the Roller Coaster, or wind vibrating pipes.
- When wind blows the pipe vibrate.
- Similar things happens with air passing through grates.

5.8 Water falling
- Water can be loud. Lowering the height water falls or decreasing the velocity can help.
- Make small adjustments and re measure.

5.9 Air Flow
Generally air creates noise by causing other things to vibrate.
- Air flows over holes to create a whistle.
- Air causes things to vibrate and create noise.
- Small changes in flow and design can make a difference.
- Check grates and air intakes.

5.10 Rattles
- These can be associated with particular speeds.
- A spectrum analysers is useful.
- Shake a suspected item to see if it makes the same noise.

5.11 Check for vibration
- A contact microphone is best.
- If no contact microphone available, hold the cell phone against the suspected source. Often the vibration will appear on the spectrum analyser

5.12 Stands that hold motors
- These can vibrate.
- The floor can also vibrate

5.13 Chutes
- Material moving along a chute can create noise.
- Lining the inside of the chute can often save money because the lining will wear first.
- This is cheaper to replace than the chute itself.

5.14 Lower the height items can fall
- Drop the item and measure.
- Make changes and measure.

5.15 Exhaust on air driven tools and rams
- Many tools have exhaust filters.
- These prevent matter entering the tool.
- Also lowers noise level.
- They can be missing or blocked.

5.16 Guards
- Often cover moving machinery.
- The movement causes Guards to make noise.

5.17 Alignment of pulleys
- If these are out of alignment noise will be created.
- Attaching a label with the recommended dB level is a good way to keep a track of wear.

5.18 large flat surfaces
- These can generate noise if something is attached to them.
- Sometimes the air pressure inside a room can tension the walls. Adjusting the room air pressure may have an effect.

5.19 Fan blades
- Dirty, worn or broken blades can generate surprising volumes of noise.
- This can also induce forced resonance and make other items in the room generate noise.

6.0 Smartphone Camera

Taking a video of noise issue is an excellent way of measuring the noise levels.

Smartphones have video capabilities

Plugging different microphones into the recording device greatly simplifies measurement.

- The sound track from the video can easily be analysed
- It can be replayed
- It can be played in slow motion
- Provides a record
- Some have built in noise level meters so sound can be seen
- The video can be sent to third parties if required.
- Easy to take more video

Choosing the right microphone is helpful.
It reduces the amount of analysis needed

> *Keeping a video is useful if noise comes and goes*
> *It provides a record that can be used in the future*

6.1 How to use Smartphone Cameras

Choose the right Microphone
 	
    i.   Directional if direction of noise needs to be found
   ii.   Contact if we suspect a surface is vibrating
  iii.   Close up if we suspect noise is coming from holes
	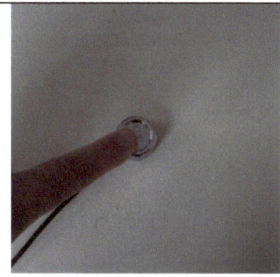
	 Contact mic used for flat surface

Plug Microphone into phone i. This by passes the camera internal Microphone	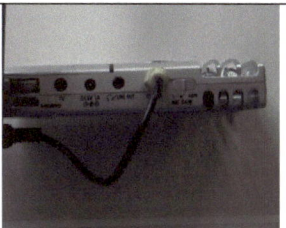

Make on camera notes
 	
    i.   Small white board
   ii.   Paper
  iii.   Post it notes
	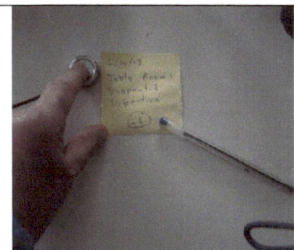

Take Video of area
 	
    i.   Slow sweeps are better
   ii. Clips of approx. 10 sec are easier to manage	

6 .2 Analyse video

Load Video into one Computer
 	
  i.   There are a number of You tube video to show how to do this
  ii. The video can be played through the computer without loading
	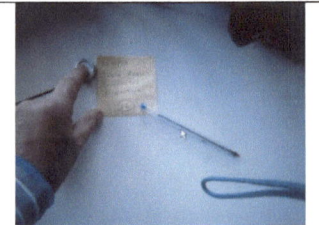

Connect Line out to Line in
 	
  i.   Line out may have an ear phone Icon
  ii. Line in may also be called Mic
	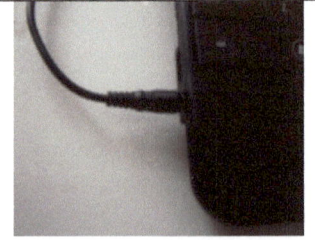

Start Spectrum analysis
 	
  i.   Start the software
  ii. Either the video can be started and stopped or the software can
	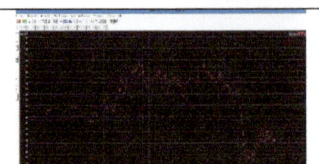

Set Up example i. The Audio on one computer goes into another	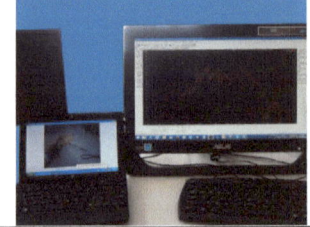

7.0 Improvement ideas

1/ Water falling
 	
    i.   Lower Height
   ii.   Make a bend in pipe
  iii.   Make a grate
  iv.   Soften landing area
	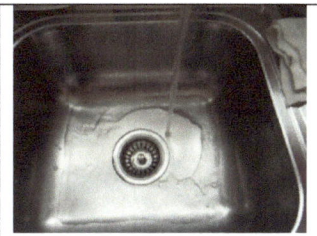

2/ Liquid entering tank
 	
    i.   Lower height
   ii.   Alter angle
  iii.   Break Flow
	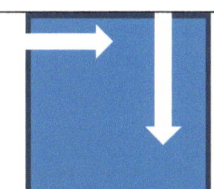

3/ Air Intakes/Exhausts
 	
    i.   The sound made can vary dependent upon the shape
   ii.   The noise made in an industrial setting has similar principle
  iii.   Measure the sound, Make alterations, measure again
	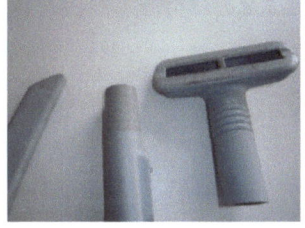

4/Whistles

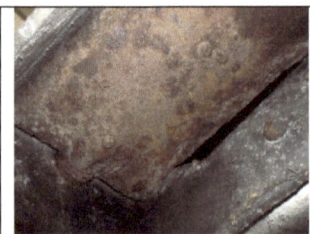

   i.   This is the air intake to a boiler
  ii.   The Flue was seized and air had worn a path.
 iii.   Freeing the flue reduced noise by 30 dB and optimised the boiler

5/ Rattles

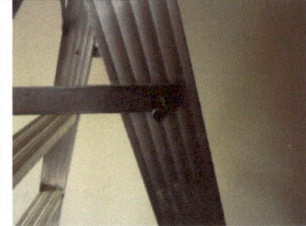

   i.   There are a number of noise sources caused by loose items
  ii.   Initially these are fixed by tightening
 iii.   The work out why they are becoming loose and eliminate

6/ Sympathetic Vibrations

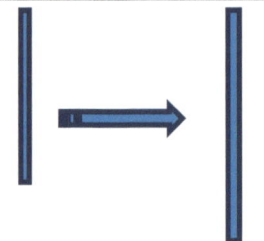

   i.   These pipes have the same resonant frequency and one causes the other to vibrate.
  ii.   Move brackets to alter frequency
 iii.   Add a little weight to break vibration
 iv.   Lag one pipe

7/ Exhaust Vents

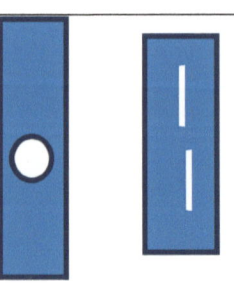

   i.   This vent had little holes
  ii.   These acted as whistles all with the same frequency
 iii.   Making slots with a grinder resolved issue
 iv.   8dB drop at Boundary of site

8/ Motors

i. This motor is rigid
ii. It causes the floor to vibrate
iii. Isolating the motor from the floor can dramatically reduce noise levels

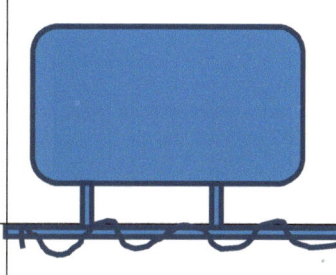

9/ Guards

i. Grid guards can vibrate
ii. They acted as a stringed instruments and whistles
iii. Replacing with a Clear guard can lower noise level

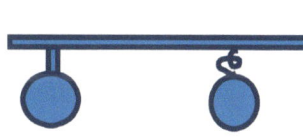

10/ Platforms acting as Drums

i. Pipes are often attached under walkways
ii. These cause the walkway to act as a drum
iii. Anchoring by using springs or rubber straps can often resolve issues

11/ Worn Pumps i. Worn pump impellers. ii. Mountings loose iii. Often the pump causes the pipes to vibrate. Lag or use springs to hold pipe.	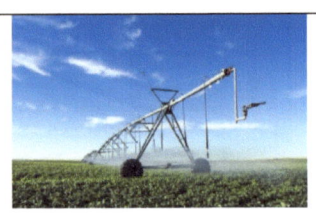
12/ Walls Acting as Drums i. The dimension of a wall makes it susceptible to act as a vibrating Membrane ii. Air variation in air pressure should be considered. iii. Check air pressure in room iv. Does it change i.e. when door opened	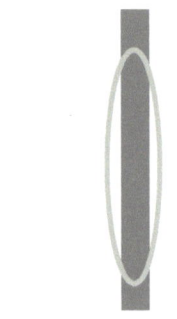
13/ Megaphone effect i. The shape of a room can act as an amplifier ii. Check the positioning of machines and move if practicable iii. Use a screen to disrupt megaphone effect	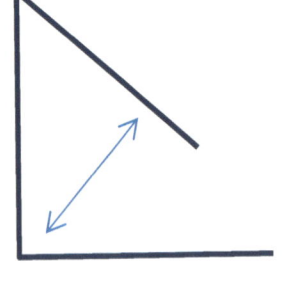

14 Liquid/Air in Pipes

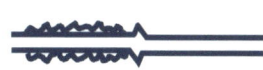

i. Air or fluid moves through Pipe
ii. The percussion of the pump or compressors generates noise and vibration inside the pipe.
iii. Noise transmits to the outside
iv. Lag pipes or fit flexible fittings
v. Expandable fittings can work very well for compressors

15 Roller Coasters

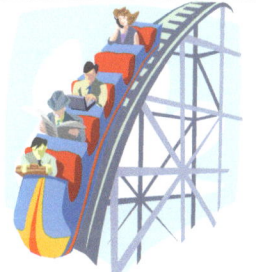

i. Wind and vibration causes the pipes to vibrate
ii. Filling rails with sand reduces noise by approx. 50%

16 Acoustic Covers

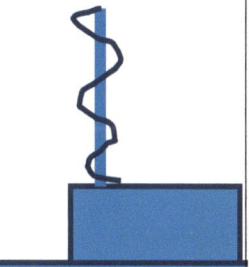

i. The cover is designed to contain noise
ii. The cover itself can create noise
iii. Often pipes entering and leaving the machine create noise.
iv. The floor may be another transmission path
v. Check paths by measuring noise

17 Worn Bearings
 	
  i.   Often Audible when machine starts and stops
  ii.   Thermal imaging cameras can pick these up.
  iii. Ultra sound will pick potential failure
  iv. A contact Microphone may pick a failure. Almost certain to register as machine stops

18/ Cavity
 	
  i.   Check for any hole or cavity
  ii.   These often build up sound and transmit it
	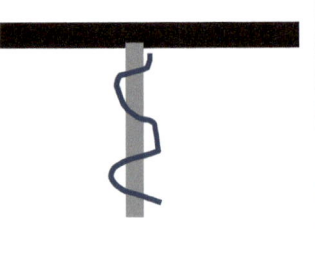

19/ Pipe supports vibrate
 	
  i.   The support for the pipe was rigid
  ii. Placing a small piece of rubber inside bracket stopped vibration	

20/ Windmill Effect

i. The windmill tower creates a vibration
ii. The vibration travels through the ground
iii. The ground then causes items attached to the ground to vibrate and create noise.
iv. Prevent the windmill tower vibrating.
v. Isolate the tower from the ground

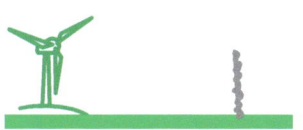

Sound can travel through the ground for over 10km dependent upon ground type

20/ Line of Sight

i. Neighbour complained about noise
ii. A vent was pointing directly at his house
iii. Redirecting vent resolved the issue

www.ingramcontent.com/pod-product-compliance
Lightning Source LLC
Chambersburg PA
CBHW041612180526
45159CB00002BC/821